Breastfeeding

Basics

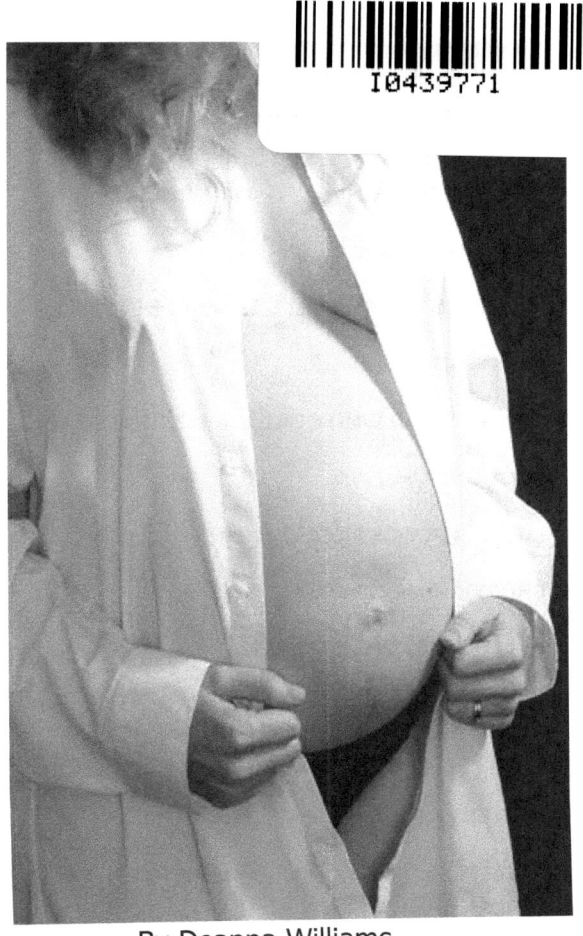

By Deanna Williams

Index

BREAST FEEDING COMPLICATIONS

HOW TO CHOOSE A BREAST PUMP

HOW TO USE A BREAST PUMP

RETURNING TO WORK

From the Author

I wrote this book because there are many misconceptions out there about breastfeeding. After personally breastfeeding both of my children I have first-hand knowledge about it. I can only hope that this book will lead you into a greater understanding of it and help you to understand all the positive benefits of it.

Yours truly,
Deanna Williams

Benefits of Breast Feeding

Once you've given birth, breast feeding is the single most important thing you can do to protect your baby and help to promote good health. Best of all, breast feeding is free.

Along with saving you money on HMR (Human Milk Replacement), breast feeding can also help you to keep your medical bills down. Babies that are fed with formula get sicker more often and more seriously than babies that are breast fed. They also have more ear infections, respiratory infections, and other problems.

This can be even more true if your family has had a history of allergies. When a baby is breast fed, the antibodies pass on from the mother to the baby, helping to protect against illness and allergies. As the baby's system matures, his body will begin to make it's own antibodies, and he'll be more equipped to handle sensitivities of food.

Sucking on the breast will also help with the development or jaw alignment and the development of the cheekbone. For this very reason, there is less of the need for costly orthodontic work when the child gets older.

Unlike formula, breast milk is always ready, always available, convenient, and always the right temperature for feeding. Plus, it contains all of the vitamins and minerals your growing baby needs, saving you a lot of money.

Breast feeding also offers many benefits for the mom as well. The baby sucking at the breast will cause contractions right after birth, leading to less bleeding for the mom, and helping her uterus to return to it's shape before pregnancy much faster.

Breast feeding will also burn calories, so a mom can lose weight much faster than if she fed her baby with a bottle. Breast feeding will also create a special bond with the mother and the baby - which is one thing formula simply cannot do.

Reasons to Breast Feed

For many years, scientists have been playing out the ingredients that make breast milk the perfect food for babies. They've discovered to day over 200 close compounds to fight infection, help the immune system mature, aid in digestion, and support brain growth - nature made properties that science simply cannot copy.

The important long term benefits of breast feeding include reduced risk of asthma, allergies, obesity, and some forms of childhood cancer. The more that scientists continue to learn, the better breast milk looks.

In addition to making your baby healthier, breast feeding may also make him smarter. Many studies have proved that breast fed babies tend to be smarter than babies who were fed with formula or other methods. Breast feeding does help with nutrients and the support of brain growth, which is something every mother should think about.

The benefits for the nursing mom are just as good as they are for the baby. The hormones that are released during breast feeding will curb blood loss post-delivery and help to shrink the uterus back to it's normal size.

Long term, the breast feeding mom will have a lower risk for pre-menopausal breast cancer, which is the kind that strikes before the age of 50. The benefits will begin to show with three to six months of breast feeding and increase the longer that breast feeding continues.

By now, you should realize that breast milk is one power packed liquid. It offers more for your baby than formula, or any other scientific creation for that matter. As you begin to plan for the future of your baby, make a commitment to breast feeding him for as long as you possibly can - as it will do both your bodies good.

Your Nursing Area

Once you've reached the third trimester, you'll probably start stocking up on nursing bras, breast pads, and loose button down shirts for the coming months ahead. Today things are so easy, you can just jump on Amazon and find all the things that you need. Check the resources section at the end of this book for some great products you will need for your baby. While getting ready to breast feed, you can also create your personal area, a custom designed breast feeding area for yourself.

Your nursing area should reflect your personality. If you like a loud, yet friendly surrounding, you should consider setting in a corner of the living room or family room. Keep an extra chair or two near you so family members or even friends can keep you company.

If you prefer peace and quiet, a cozy study or empty guest room would be ideal. You can close the door, dim the lights down, then take a few deep, calming breaths while you breast feed.

Your own chair

No matter if it's a glider, overstuffed recliner, or desk chair with wheels, you should make sure your nursing chair is very comfortable. You'll be sitting in the chair for hours each day, so you'll want it to be very comfortable. You should always look for one that offers back and shoulder support, along with arm rests.

Support underfoot

You can use a footstool, low coffee table or a stack of pillows to elevate your feet as you breast feed. If you raise your legs and feet to bring your baby to your breast, you'll avoid possible backache.

Pillows and more pillows

Your neck, arms, feet, and back will need as much support as you can give, so don't hesitate to surround your body with pillows. If you lay a pillow across your lap for your baby to lay on, he'll be very comfortable and that much closer to your nipple. For extra comfort, you can even purchase a specially made nursing pillow that will encircle your waist.

Table for one

You should always keep a small table or stand within arm's length of your breast feeding chair. What you use should be big enough to hold a coaster and glass of liquid. Some women prefer to drink through a straw, while others prefer to drink from the glass.

You'll also want to keep healthy snacks on hand as well, such as fresh fruit, nuts, or crackers and peanut butter to help you replace the energy you use while you breast feed.

Distractions

If your baby is a slow eater or has a really big appetite, you may want to keep yourself busy while he feeds. You can fill the shelves of a nearby cupboard or bookcase with your favorite books or crossword puzzles to occupy yourself until your baby is full. You should also keep a phone nearby as well so that you can talk to family or friends to pass the time.

Refusal to Breast Feed

Sometimes, a baby that is breast fed may suddenly decide to refuse breast feeding. The baby will pull away from the breast, then toss his head from side to side. This can happen at anytime, so there really is no way to predict it happening.

Reasons why

Refusal to feed from the breast could occur when the baby is in pain. Normally, this can be due to an ear infection, sore head from vacuum delivery, thrush in the baby's mouth, or teething.

The use of dummies, teats or nipple shields may also contribute to refusal. Some babies actually find it difficult to feed from the breast and bottle as the sucking action is very different. Some become confused, therefore it's always best to avoid using any type of teats or dummies.

Sometimes, the milk just tastes bitter. This can be due to antibiotics, if you starting or in the middle of your period, or nipple creams. If the milk tastes bitter, your baby will normally not want to feed.

Solving the problems

First, you should always try to identify what may have caused the breast refusal then begin to treat the cause. Always remain patient and gentle with your baby. Be sure to hold your baby next to you, skin to skin, so that he can take the breast when he wants to, so that he begins to realize that breast feeding is both enjoyable and comfortable.

Older babies may suddenly take shorter and fewer breast feeds, although this can be normal with some babies. Therefore, it's always best not to try and make the baby feed longer, but instead let the baby decide how often and also how long each individual feeding will last.

How Breast Milk is Made

If you've ever been pregnant or if you are pregnant now, you've probably noticed a metamorphosis in your bra cups. The physical changes (tender, swollen breasts) may be one of the earliest clues that you have conceived. Many experts believe that the color change in the areola may also be helpful when it comes to breast feeding.

What's going on

Perhaps what's even more remarkable than visible changes is the extensive changes that are taking place inside of your breasts. The developing placenta stimulates the release of estrogen and progesterone, which will in turn stimulate the complex biological system that helps to make lactation possible.

Before you get pregnant, a combination of supportive tissue, milk glands, and fat make up the larger portions of your breasts. The fact is, your newly swollen breasts have been preparing for your pregnancy since you were in your mother's womb!

When you were born, your main milk ducts had already formed. Your mammary glands stayed quiet until you reached puberty, when a flood of the female hormone estrogen caused them to grow and also to swell. During pregnancy, those glands will kick into high gear.

Before your baby arrives, glandular tissue has replaced a majority of the fat cells and accounts for your bigger than before breasts. Each breast may actually get as much as 1 1/2 pounds heavier than before!

Nestled among the fatty cells and glandular tissue is an intricate network of channels or canals known as the milk ducts. The pregnancy hormones will cause these ducts to increase in both number and size, with the ducts branching off into smaller canals near the chest wall known as ductiles.

At the end of each duct is a cluster of smaller sacs known as alveoli. The cluster of alveoli is known as a lobule, while a cluster of lobule is known as a lobe. Each breast will contain around 15 - 20 lobes, with one milk duct for every lobe.

The milk is produced inside of the alveoli, which is surrounded by tiny muscles that squeeze the glands and help to push the milk out into the ductiles. Those ductiles will lead to a bigger duct that widens into a milk pool directly below the areola.

The milk pools will act as reservoirs that hold the milk until your baby sucks it through the tiny openings in your nipples. Mother Nature is so smart that your milk duct system will become fully developed around the time of your second trimester, so you can properly breast feed your baby even if he or she arrives earlier than you are anticipating.

Getting Started With Breast Feeding

When you hold your baby for the first time in the delivery room, you should put his lips to your breast. Although your mature milk hasn't developed yet, your breasts are still producing a substance known as colostrum that helps to protect your baby from infections.

If your baby has trouble finding or staying on your nipple, you shouldn't panic. Breast feeding is an art that will require a lot of patience and a lot of practice. No one expects you to be an expert when you first start, so you shouldn't hesitate to ask for advice or have a nurse show you what you need to do.

Once you start, keep in mind that nursing shouldn't be painful. When your baby latches on, pay attention to how your breasts feel. If the latching on hurts, break the suction then try again.

You should nurse quite frequently, as the more you nurse the more quickly your mature milk will come in and the more milk you'll produce. Breast feeding for 10 - 15 minutes per breast 8 - 10 times every 24 hours is an ideal target. Crying is a sign of hunger, which means you should actually feed your baby before he starts crying.

During the first few days, you may have to wake your baby to begin breast feeding, and he may end up falling asleep during feeding. To ensure that your baby is eating often enough, you should wake him up if it has been four hours since the last time he has been fed.

Getting comfortable

Feedings can take 40 minutes or longer, therefore you'll want a cozy spot. You don't want to be sitting somewhere where you will be bothered, as it can make the process very hard.

The First Six Weeks

Breast milk is the best food you can give to your baby. Breast milk is a complete food source, containing all the nutrients your baby need – at least 400 of them to be exact, including hormones and disease fighting compounds that aren't found in formula.

The nutritional makeup in breast milk will adjust to your baby's needs as he or she grows and develops. Aside from the brain building, infection fighting benefits of breast milk, which no formula can match, nursing will also help to build a special bond between you and your baby. When nursing, your child thrives on the contact, cuddling, and holding - which you will as well.

Since breast feedings can take up to 40 minutes or more, you should pick a cozy spot for nursing. The atmosphere is very important, even more so in the early days of breast feeding when you're still trying to get the hang of it. If you get easily distracted by noise, go somewhere quiet.

You should always hold your baby in a position that won't leave your arms or back sore. It works the best to support the back of your baby's head with your hand, although which position you choose depends on what's more comfortable to you.

When supporting your baby, a nursing pillow can sometimes be a big help. You should never feed until both you and your baby are comfortable. Pay attention to how your breasts feel when your baby latches on, as his mouth should cover most of the areola below the nipple, and the nipple should be far back into your baby's mouth.

While some women adjust to breast feeding easily, other moms find it hard to learn. If you feel discouraged, always know that you aren't the only one. Everyone feels different when starting, it all depends on the mother and the situation.

Breast feeding will take practice. Therefore, you should give yourself as much time as you need to get it down to second nature. Always take it one feeding at a time. If you are having a bad day, tell yourself that it'll get better. Keep in mind that any problems are temporary, as you'll be nursing like a pro by your six week postpartum checkup.

The first six weeks will be both an adventure and training. You can't expect to know everything when you begin, which is where training and practice will really help you excel. The more you breast feed, the more you'll learn. You'll also build a bond with your baby - which is something you'll always have for the rest of your lives.

Breast Feeding and Positioning

For some people, the process of breast feeding seems to come natural, although there's a level of skill required for successful feeding and a correct technique to use. Incorrect positioning is one of the biggest reasons for unsuccessful feeding and it can even injure the nipple or breast quite easily.

By stroking the baby's cheek with the nipple, the baby will open its mouth towards the nipple, which should then be pushed in so that the baby will get a mouthful of nipple and areola. This position is known as latching on. A lot of women prefer to wear a nursing bra to allow easier access to the breast than other normal bras.

The length of feeding time will vary. Regardless of the duration of feeding time, it's important for mothers to be comfortable. The following are positions you can use:

1. Upright - The sitting position where the back is straight.

2. Mobile - Mobile is where the mother carries her baby in a sling or carrier while breast feeding. Doing this allows the mother to breast feed in the work of everyday life.

3. Lying down - This is good for night feeds or for those who have had a caesarean section.

4. On her back - The mother is sitting slightly upright, also a useful position for tandem breast feeding.

5. On her side - The mother and baby both lie on their sides.

6. Hands and knees - In this feeding position the mother is on all fours with the baby underneath her. Keep in mind, this position isn't normally recommended.

Anytime you don't feel comfortable with a feeding position, always stop and switch to a different position. Each position is different, while some mothers prefer one position, other's may like a totally different position. All you need to do is experiment and see which position is best for you.

Engorged Breasts

Within the first two to three days after you have iven birth, you may discover that your breasts feel swollen, tender, throbbing, lumpy, and overly full. Sometimes, the swelling will extend all the way to your armpit, and you may run a low fever as well.

The causes

Within 72 hours of giving birth, an abundance of milk will come in or become available to your baby. As this happens, more blood will flow o your breasts and some of the surrounding tissue will swell. The result is full, swollen, engorged breasts.

Not every postpartum mom experienced true engorgement. Some women's breasts become only slightly full, while others find their breasts have become amazingly hard. Some women will hardly notice the pain, as they are involved in other things during the first few days.

Treating it

Keep in mind, engorgement is a positive sign that you are producing milk to feed to your baby. Until you produce the right amount:

1. Wear a supportive nursing bra, even at night - making sure it isn't too tight.

2. Breast feed often, every 2 - 3 hours if you can. Try to get the first side of your breasts as soft as possible. If your baby seems satisfied with just one breast, you can offer the other at the next feeding.

3. Avoid letting your baby latch on and suck when the areola is very firm. To reduce the possibility of nipple damage, you can use a pump until your areola softens up.

4. Avoid pumping milk except when you need to soften the areola or when your baby is unable to latch on. Excessive pumping can lead to the over production of milk and prolonged engorgement.

5. To help soothe the pain and relieve swelling, apply cold packs to your breasts for a short amount of time after you nurse. Crushed ice in a plastic bag will also work.

6. Look ahead. You'll get past this engorgement in no time and soon be able to enjoy your breast feeding relationship with your new baby.

Engorgement will pass very quickly. You can expect it to diminish within 24 - 48 hours, as nursing your baby will only help the problem. If you aren't breast feeding, it will normally get worse before it gets better. Once the engorgement has passed, your breasts will be softer and still full of milk.

During this time, you can and should continue to nurse. Unrelieved engorgement can cause a drop in your production of milk, so it's important to breast feed right from the start. Keep an eye for signs of hunger and feed him when he needs to be fed.

Avoiding Foods While Breast Feeding

Many women find that they can eat whatever they may like during breast feeding. Even though it's true that some strongly favored foods can change the taste of your milk, many babies seem to enjoy the varieties of breast milk flavors. Occasionally, your baby may get cranky at the breast after you eat certain foods. If you notice this happening, simply avoid that particular food.

The most common offenders during breast feeding include chocolate, spices, citrus fruits, garlic, chili, lime, gassy vegetables, and fruits with laxative type effects, such as prunes and cherries.

You can have a cup or two of coffee a day, although too much caffeine can interfere with your baby's sleep and even make him or her cranky. Keep in mind, caffeine is found in many soda's, tea, and even over the counter type medicine as well.

It's okay to have an alcoholic beverage every now and the, although having more than one drink can increase your blood alcohol level, putting the alcohol into your breast milk.

If you are planning to have more than one drink at a time, it's best to wait two hours or more per drink before you resume any type of nursing or breast feeding. There is no need to pump and dump unless your breasts are full and its time to feed your baby. While breast feeding, any type of heavy drinking should be avoided.

Before you actually omit any foods from your diet, you should talk to your doctor. If you avoid certain foods and it causes a nutritional imbalance, you may need to see a nutritionist for advice on taking other foods or getting nutritional supplements.

Health and Diet

The nutritional requirements for the baby will rely soley on the breast milk, and therefore the mother will need to maintain a healthy diet. If the baby is large and grows fast, the fat stores gained by the mother during pregnancy can be depleted quickly, meaning that she may have trouble eating good enough to maintain and develop sufficient amounts of milk.

This type of diet normally involves a high calorie, high nutrition diet which follows on from that in pregnancy. Even though mothers in famine conditions can produce milk with nutritional content, a mother that is malnourished may produce milk with lacking levels of vitamins A, D, B6, and B12.

If they smoke, breast feeding mothers must use extreme caution. More than 20 cigarettes a day has been shown to reduce the milk supply and cause vomiting, diarrhoea, rapid heart rate, and restlessness in the infants. SIDS (Sudden Infant Death Syndrome) is more common in babies that are exposed to smoke.

Heavy drinking is also known to harm the infant, as well as yourself. If you are breast feeding, you should avoid alcohol or consume very small amounts at a time.

The excessive consumption of alcohol by the mother can result in irritability, sleeplessness, and increased feeding in the infant. Moderate use, normally 1 – 2 cups a day normally produces no effect. Therefore, mothers that are breast feeding are advised to avoid caffeine or restrict intake of it.

By following a healthy diet and limiting your intake of the above, you'll ensure that your baby gets the right nutrients during your time of breast feeding.

This stage of life is very important - as you don't want anything to happen to your baby.

Other Foods While Breast Feeding

Breast milk is actually the only food your baby will need until 4 months of age, although most babies do well on breast milk alone for 6 months or better. There is really no advantage to adding other foods or milks before 4 - 6 months, except under unusual circumstances.

Water

Breast milk is over 90% water. Even in the hottest days of summer, a baby won't require any extra water. If a baby isn't feeding well, they still don't require any extra water – although they will need the breast feeding problems to be fixed.

Vitamin D

Although breast milk doesn't contain much vitamin D, it does have a little. The baby will store up vitamin D during pregnancy, and remain healthy without any vitamin D supplementation, unless you yourself had a problem with vitamin D deficiency when pregnant.

Exposure to the outside will give your baby vitamin D, even in winter and when the sky is covered. An hour or more exposure during the week will give your baby more than enough vitamin D.

Iron

Breast milk contains less iron than formulas do, especially those that are iron enriched. Iron will give the baby added protection against infections, as many bacteria need iron in order to multiply.

The iron found in breast milk is utilized well by the baby, while not being available to bacteria. The introduction of iron should never be delayed beyond the age of 6 months.

Breast milk is the best that you can feed your baby, as it provides everything he will need for probably the first 6 months. After the first 6 months, you can introduce solid foods to your baby if he is taking an interest to them.

Poor Milk Supply

Almost all women don't have a problem with producing enough milk to breast feed. The ideal way to make sure that your baby is getting enough milk is to be sure that he's well positioned, attached to the breast, and feed him as often as he gets hungry.

Some mom's that are breast feeding will stop before they want to, simply because they don't think they have enough breast milk.

There are signs that might make you believe your baby isn't getting enough milk. If your baby seems hungry or unsettled after feeding, or if he wants to feed often with short pauses between feedings, you may think he isn't getting enough milk - which are often times not the case.

There are however, two reliable signs that let you know your baby isn't getting enough milk. If your baby has poor or really slow weight gain, or is passing small amounts of concentrated urine, he's not getting enough milk.

All babies will lose weight within the first few days after birth. Babies are born with supplies of fat and fluids, which will help them keep going for the first several days.

Once your baby regains birth weight, he should begin putting on around 200g for the first four months or so. To get back to their birth weight, it normally takes a few weeks.

If the weight gain for your baby seems to be slow, don't hesitate to ask your doctor or nurse to observe you breast feeding. This way, they can make sure that your technique is right and if they think your baby is breast feeding often enough.

To help you with your breast feeding, here are some ways that you can increase your supply of milk:

1. Be sure that your baby is positioned correctly and attached to your breast.

2. Let your baby feed for as long and often as he wants.

3. If you feel that your baby isn't breast feeding enough, offer him more breast feeds.

4. During each breast feed, make sure you feed from both breasts.

5. If your baby has been using a dummy, make sure you stop him.

6. Some babies may be sleepy and reluctant to feed, which may be the cause of problems with milk supply.

By following the above tips, you'll do your part in making sure you have enough milk when it comes time to breast feed. If you are uncertain or have other questions, be sure to ask your doctor, as he can answer any type of question you may have.

Low Supply Of Breast Milk

Almost all mothers who breast feed go through a period of questioning whether or not their supply of milk is adequate. Some mothers simply aren't able to produce enough milk to meet the needs of her baby. According to many experts, true insufficiencies of milk are very rare.

A lot of women think their milk supply is low when it actually isn't. Thinking this can happen if you lose the feeling of fullness in your breasts or if the milk stops leaking from your nipples. Babies that go through growth spurts may want more milk than usual, and these more frequent feedings may leave your breasts less than full.

Causes of it

A mother's milk supply may diminish for a brief period of time if she isn't feeding her baby often enough due to nipple pain, or a poor latch on technique. Illnesses or estrogen containing birth control pills may also affect the production of milk.

What you should do

The best way to handle a low supply of breast milk is through a doctor's care. You should make sure that your baby gets frequent feedings and that nothing is wrong with your nipples or your milk ducts. Doctors are the best ones to ask, as they can run tests to see if everything is fine within your body.

A low supply of breast milk can affect your baby, although it's more of a mental condition than anything else. If your baby isn't gaining any weight or if he is losing weight, you should call a doctor immediately. Improved techniques for breast feeding will normally help, although in some cases weight gain or weight loss will indicate a serious concern.

In most cases, you can still nurse with a temporary decrease in milk supply, although frequent breast feeding is the key to boosting your production of milk.

Breast Compression

The sole purpose of breast compression is to continue the flow of milk to the baby once the baby no longer drinks on his own. Compression will also stimulate a let down reflex and often causes a natural let down reflex to occur. This technique may also be useful for the following:

1. Poor weight gain in the baby.

2. Colic in the breast fed baby.

3. Frequent feedings or long feedings.

4. Sore nipples for the mother.

5. Recurrent blocked ducts

6. Feeding the baby who falls asleep quick.

If everything is going well, breast compression may not be necessary. When all is well, the mother should allow the baby to finish feeding on the first side, then if the baby wants more - offer the other side.

How to use breast compression :

1. Hold the baby with one arm.

2. Hold the breast with the other arm, thumb on one side of your breast, your finger on the other far back from the nipple

3. Keep an eye out for the baby's drinking, although there is no need to be obsessive about catching every suck. The baby will get more milk when drinking with an open pause type of suck.

4. When the baby is nibbling or no longer drinking, compress the breast, not so hard that it hurts though. With the breast compression, the baby should begin drinking again.

5. Keep up the pressure until the baby no longer drinks with the compression, then release the pressure. If the baby doesn't stop sucking with the release of compression, wait a bit before compressing again.

6. The reason for releasing pressure is to allow your hand to rest, and allow the milk to begin flowing to the baby again. If the baby stops sucking when you release the pressure, he'll start again once he tastes milk.

7. When the baby starts to suck again, he may drink. If not, simply compress again.

8. Continue feeding on the first side until the baby no longer drinks with compression. You should allow him time to stay on that side until he starts drinking again, on his own.

9. If the baby is no longer drinking, allow to come off the breast or take him off.

10. If the baby still wants more, offer the other side and repeat the process as above.

11. Unless you have sore nipples, you may want to switch sides like this several times.

12. Always work to improve the baby's latch.

Breast Feeding in Public

Babies that are breast fed are very portable and easy to comfort no matter where your schedule has you going. Many women however, worry about breast feeding in public. The worry of nursing in a public place is normally worse than the actual experience and often times the only people who notice you feeding are the other mothers who are doing the same thing.

Many women find ways to breast feed discreetly. You can ask your partner or even a friend to stand in front of you while you lift your shirt from the waist. When you breast feed, the baby's body will cover most of your upper body and you can pull your shirt down to her face to cover the tops of your breast. Some mothers prefer to put a light blanket over their shoulders as a type of cover.

When you are visiting someone else's home, you may feel more comfortable either leaving the room or turning away from people when you first put the baby to your breast. If you would like more privacy, breast feed in an empty room, car, or public restroom.

A lot of restrooms are becoming more baby friendly and they even have a separate are with a changing table and a chair. Several shopping malls now offer special mother's rooms where the mom can breast feed her baby in privacy, which will help sensitive babies who are too distracted by feeding to nurse well in public. It won't take long at all though, before your baby will learn to breast feed without any fuss at all.

An alternative way is expressing or pumping your milk at home and then offer it in a bottle while in public. Keep in mind, offering bottles with artificial nipples in the first few weeks can and probably will interfere with breast feeding.

When breast feeding in public, you should always use what works best for you. During the first few weeks, it will take some getting used to, as it will be as new for you as it is for the baby. With some time, you'll have no problems at all.

If you don't feel comfortable breast feeding in a certain location, then you shouldn't. You should feel a certain level of comfort when you feed, as the baby can tell when you aren't comfortable doing something. If you show your baby that you aren't nervous - you and your baby will be just fine.

Weaning From Breast Feeding

When your baby has stopped breast feeding and gets all of his nutrition from other sources than the breast, he's actually considered weaned. Even though babies are also weaned from the bottle as well, the term weaning often refers to when a baby is stopped from breast feeding.

When weaning is a mother's idea, it normally requires a lot of patience and can take time, depending on the age of your baby or toddler, and also how well your child adjusts. The overall experience is different for everyone.

Weaning is a long goodbye, sometimes emotional and sometimes painful. It doesn't however, signal of the end to the intimacy you and your child have developed during the nursing stage. What it means, is that you have to replace breast feeding with other types of nourishment.

Starting weaning

Your the best judge as to when it's the right time to wean, and you don't really have a deadline unless you and your child are actually ready to wean. The recommended time for weaning is one year. No matter what relatives, friends, or even complete strangers tell you, there is no right or wrong time for weaning.

How to wean

You should proceed slowly, regardless of what the age of your child may be. Experts say that you shouldn't abruptly withhold your breast, as they results can be traumatic. You should however, try these methods instead:

1. Skip a feeding - Skip a feeding and see what happens, offering a cup of milk to your baby instead. As a substitute, you can use a bottle of your own pumped milk, formula, or a cow's milk. If you reduce feedings one at a time, your child will eventually adjust to the changes.

2. Shorten feeding time - You can start by cutting the length of time your child is actually at the breast. If the normal feeding time is 5 minutes, try 3. Depending on the age, follow the feeding with a healthy snack. Bed time feedings are usually the hardest to wean, as they are normally the last to go.

3. Postpone and distract - You can postpone feedings if you are only feeding a couple of times per day. This method works great if you have an older child you can actually reason with. If your child wants the breast, say that you'll feed later then distract him. If you've tried everything and weaning doesn't seem to be working at all, maybe the time just isn't right. You can wait just a bit longer to see what happens, as your child and you have to determine the right time to wean together.

Breast Feeding Toddlers

Because more and more women are choosing to breast feed their babies, more and more are also finding that they enjoy it enough to continue longer than the first few months they planned on. Breast feeding to 3 - 4 years of age is common in much of the world recently, and is still common in many societies for toddlers to be breast fed.

Because mothers and babies often enjoy to breast feed, you shouldn't stop it. After six months, many think that breast milk loses it's value - which isn't true. Even after six months, it still contains protein, fat, and other important nutrients which babies and children need.

The fact is, immune factors in breast milk will protect the baby against infections. Breast milk also contains factors that will help the immune system mature, and other organs to develop and mature as well.

It's been shown and proven in the past that children in daycare who are still breast feeding have far less severe infections than the children that aren't breast feeding. The mother will lose less work time if she chooses to continue nursing her baby once she is back to work.

If you have thought about breast feeding your baby once he gets past 6 months of age, you have made a wise decision. Although many feel that it isn't necessary, breast milk will always help babies and toddlers. Breast milk is the best milk you can give to your baby.

No matter what others may tell you, breast feeding only needs to be stopped when you and the baby agree on it. You don't have to stop when someone else wants you to - you should only stop when you feel that it's the right time.

Starting Solid Foods

Breast milk is all your baby will need until at least 4 months of age. There does come a time, when breast milk will no longer supply all of your baby's nutrition needs. Full term babies will start to require iron from other sources by 6 – 9 months of age.

Some babies that aren't started on solid foods by the age of 9 - 12 months may have a great level of difficulty accepting solid foods. It's actually a developmental milestone when your child starts solid foods - as he is now growing up.

When to start

The ideal time to begin solid foods is when the baby shows interest in starting. Some babies will show interest in solid food when it's on their parents' plates, as early as 4 months of age. By 5 - 6 months, most babies will reach out and try to grab the food. When the baby starts to reach for food, it's normally the time to go ahead and give him some.

Sometimes, it may be a better idea to start food earlier. When a baby seems to get hungry or once weight gain isn't continuing at the desired rate, it may be good to start solid foods as early as 3 months. It may be possible however, to continue breast feeding alone and have the baby less hungry or growing more rapidly.

Breast fed babies will digest solid foods better and earlier than artificially fed babies because the breast milk will contain enzymes which help to digest fats, proteins, and starch. Breast fed babies will also have had a variety of different tastes in their life, since the flavors of many foods the mother eats will pass into her milk.

Introducing solid foods

When the baby begins to take solid foods at the age of 5 - 6 months, there is very little difference what he starts will or what order it is introduced. You should however, avoid spicy foods or highly allergenic foods at first, although if your baby reaches for the potato on your plate, you should let him have it if it isn't too hot.

Offer your baby the foods that he seems to be interested in. Allow your baby to enjoy the food and don't worry too much about how much he takes at first, as much of it may end up on the floor or in his hair anyhow.

The easiest way to get iron for your baby at 5 - 6 months of age is by giving him meat. Cereal for infants has iron, although it is poorly absorbed and may cause your baby to get constipated.

Breast Feeding Adopted Babies

Not only is breast feeding an adopted baby easy, the chances are that you will produce a large amount of milk. It isn't complicated to do, although it is different than breast feeding a baby you have been pregnant with for 9 months.

Breast feeding and milk

There are two objectives that are involved in breast feeding an adopted baby. The first is getting your baby to breast feed, and the other is producing enough breast milk.

There is more to breast feeding than just milk, which is why many mothers are happy to feed without expecting to produce milk in the way the baby needs. It's the closeness and the bond breast feeding provides that many mothers look for.

Taking the breast

Even though many feel the early introduction of bottles may interfere with breast feeding, the early introduction of artificial nipples can interfere a great deal. The sooner you can get the baby to the breast after birth, the better things will be.

Babies will however, require the flow from the breast in order to stay attached and continue to suck, especially if they are used to getting flow from a bottle or other method of feeding.

Producing breast milk

As soon as you have an adopted baby in sight, contact a lactation clinic and start getting your milk supply ready. Keep in mind, you may never produce a full milk supply for your baby, although it may happen. You should never feel discouraged by what you may be pumping before the baby, as a pump is never quite as good at extracting milk as a baby who is well latched and sucking.

Breast Feeding and Jaundice

Jaundice is a result of buildup in the blood of the bilirubin, a yellow pigment that comes from the breakdown of older red blood cells. It's normal for the red blood cells to break down, although the bilirubin formed doesn't normally cause jaundice because the liver will metabolize it and then get rid of it in the gut.

However, the newborn baby will often become jaundiced during the first few days due to the liver enzyme that metabolizes the bilirubin becoming relatively immature. Therefore, newborn babies will have more red blood cells than adults, and thus more will break down at any given time.

Breast milk jaundice

There is a condition that's commonly referred to as breast milk jaundice, although no one knows what actually causes it. In order to diagnose it, the baby should be at least a week old. The baby should also be gaining well with breast feeding alone, having lots of bowel movements with the passing of clean urine.

In this type of setting, the baby has what is referred to as breast milk jaundice. On occasion, infections of the urine or an under functioning of the baby's thyroid gland, as well as other rare illnesses that may cause the same types of problems.

Breast milk jaundice will peak at 10 - 21 days, although it can last for 2 - 3 months. Contrary to what you may think, breast milk jaundice is normal. Rarely, if at all ever, does breast feeding need to be stopped for even a brief period of time.

If the baby is doing well on breast milk, there is no reason at all to stop or supplement with a lactation aid.

Breast Feeding Complications

Sore nipples

A lot of mothers complain about tender nipples that make breast feeding painful and frustrating. There is good news though, as most mothers don't suffer that long. The nipples will toughen up quickly and render breast feeding virtually painless.

Improperly positioned babies or babies that suck really hard can make the breasts extremely sore. Below, are some ways to ease your discomfort:

1. Make sure your baby is in the correct position, since a baby that isn't positioned correctly is the number one cause of sore nipples.

2. Once you have finished feeding, expose your breasts to the air and try to protect them from clothing and other irritations.

3. After breast feeding, apply some ultra purified, medical grade lanolin, making sure to avoid petroleum jelly and other products with oil.

4. Make sure to wash your nipples with water and not with soap.

5. Many women find teabags ran under cold water to provide some relief when placed on the nipples.

6. Make sure you vary your position each time with feeding to ensure that a different area of the nipple is being compressed each time.

Clogged milk ducts

Clogged milk ducts can be identified as small, red tender lumps on the tissue of the breast. Clogged ducts can cause the milk to back up and lead to infection. The best way to unclog these ducts is to ensure that you've emptied as completely as possible. You should offer the clogged breast first at feeding time, then let your baby empty it as much as possible.

If milk remains after the feeding, the remaining amount should be removed by hand or with a pump. You should also keep pressure off the duct by making sure your bra is not too tight.

Breast infection

Also known as mastititis, breast infection is normally due to empty breasts completely out of milk, germs gaining entrance to the milk ducts through cracks or fissures in the nipple, and decreased immunity in the mother due to stress or inadequate nutrition.

The symptoms of breast infection include severe pain or soreness, hardness of the breast, redness of the breast, heat coming from the area, swelling, or even chills.

The treatment of breast infection includes bed rest, antibiotics, pain relievers, increased fluid intake, and applying heat. Many women will stop breast feeding during an infection, although it's actually the wrong thing to do. By emptying the breasts, you'll actually help to prevent clogged milk ducts.

If the pain is so bad you can't feed, try using a pump while laying in a tub of warm water with your breasts floating comfortably in the water. You should also make sure that the pump isn't electric if you plan to use it in the bath tub.

You should always make sure that breast infections are treated promptly and completely or you may risk the chance of abscess. An abscess is very painful, involving throbbing and swelling. You'll also experience swelling, tenderness, and heat in the area of the abscess. If the infection progresses this far, your doctor may prescribe medicine and even surgery.

How to Choose A Breast Pump

The milk production in the breasts, much like so many other things, work on the shear principal of supply and demand. The more breast milk your baby consumes, the more your body will need to make.

Breast pumps are generally used to insure continued production of breast milk when you cannot feed your baby - whether you are back to work, traveling, taking medication, or just out of town.

Basic types of pumps

Breast pumps can either be battery operated, hand operated, semi automatic electric, or even self cycling electric.

Hand pumps

Manual hand pumps are designed to use the strength of your hand or arm muscles for pumping one breast at a time. You can also get pumps that will use the leg and foot muscles for pumping both breasts at one time. Mothers that with carpal tunnel syndrome may want to consider using a pump designed for the arm or leg muscles or even an automatic model.

Battery operated pumps

Pumps with battery operation are the best for women who have an established supply of milk and want to pump once or even twice a day. These pumps use batteries to create suction, minimizing any type of muscle fatigue. Most battery type pumps are designed for pumping one breast at a time and are recommended for occasional usage.

Electric pumps

Even though electric pumps are more efficient than hand or even battery operated pumps, they also tend to be more expensive. You can however, rent them if you need to. Electric pumps can normally plug directly into an outlet and are designed for pumping both breasts at a time and even frequent use. Hospital grade pumps are the most efficient for initiating and maintaining milk supply, and are available for rent or purchase.

How to Use A Breast Pump

Just like breast feeding, pumping is a skill that you learn. When first trying a breast pump, most mothers are only able to express a few drops of milk. With the proper practice and knowledge, the mother will be more efficient at pumping.

Preparing the breast pump

1. Read all the instructions in the kit very carefully.

2. Every part of the breast pump will need to be sterilized before you begin using it.

3. After use, all the parts of the pump will need to be washed in warm, soapy water, then rinsed with hot water and drained on a clean towel. The plastic tubing doesn't need to be cleaned unless you get milk into it. If you do wash it, it should be hung to allow time to dry and drain thoroughly.

4. If your doctor feels the need, the entire kit can be sterilized every day.

5. When you first start with an electric pump, the suction level should be on the lowest possible setting.

Getting started

- Warm compresses, gentle massages of the breast and gentle nipple stimulation will help to stimulate a quick let down.

- You should always relax while doing breast massages during pumping. Some mothers prefer to close their eyes then think about nursing the baby, imagining the baby in their arms. The more relaxed a mother is, the better let down she'll have and the more milk will be dispensed.

- Your first attempts at pumping should be considered practice sessions with learning to use the breast pump as the goal, not how much milk is actually dispensed.

- When you use a hand pump, quick, short pumps at the start is stimulating and will imitate more closely the way a baby breast feeds. Once the let down occurs and milk starts to flow freely, long, steadier strokes are more effective and less tiring.

-   When you learn to pump, you should practice for 5 minutes on a side at least once or twice a day. Always pick the least stressful part of your day for pumping.

Relaxing and realizing that the pump is your friend is the single most important thing that a mother can do. There are several things that a mother can do to help herself relax, such as putting a picture of the baby on the pump, playing cards or a game with friends, watching television, read books, or talk on the phone. Simply watching the collection bottle is not helpful and will probably put more stress on you than you actually need.

Returning To Work

Once you return to work, you can continue to breast feed. If you live close to work or have an on site daycare, you may be able to breast feed during your breaks. If that isn't possible, you have 2 choices:

1. Keep your milk supply by using a high quality automatic electric breast pump to express milk during the day. Save your milk that you collect for your baby sitter.

2. If you don't want to or can't pump at work, you can gradually replace daytime feedings with formula while you're at home but still continue to nurse at night and in the morning. The milk your body produces may not be enough to keep your baby satisfied, even if you only need enough for 2 feedings.

Advantages of pumping at work

Pumping at work will help stimulate your production of milk, so you'll have plenty available when it comes time to feed. You can also collect the milk you pump, so your baby will have the health and nutritional benefits of breast milk even when you aren't there. To make things better, pumping can be an ideal way to feel a connection to your baby during the work day.

Although it can seem like a hassle, many mothers find that the benefits of breast pumping far outweigh the inconvenience.

To manage pumping at work, you'll need to have the following:

1. Breast pump, preferably a fully automatic electric pump with a double collection kit so you can pump both breasts simultaneously.

2. Bottles or bags for collecting and storing the milk.

3. Access to a refrigerator or cooler to keep the milk cold until you return home.

4. Breast pads to help protect your clothes if you start to leak. (see resources page)

Make sure that you get used to pumping before you return to work, so you'll know what to expect and how it feels. You'll be much more confident with pumping at work if you already know that you can produce enough milk.

At work, you'll want to have somewhere that's away from everyone else when you pump, such as an empty office or empty room. This way, you'll be away from everyone else and you can have the quiet tranquility you need to pump. In most offices, this shouldn't be a problem.

For the time frame, you'll want to pump every 2 - 3 hours if possible. (If you can't, every 4 hours or so will have to suffice.) After you have finished pumping, store the milk in the bags or bottles, clean yourself up, then go back to work. When you return home, you can feed the milk to your growing baby.

Resources

None of these are affiliate links, just links to some really great products for your new baby.

Nursing pads
http://amzn.com/B00Q75D7VQ

Charcoal Bamboo inserts for cloth diapers
http://amzn.com/B00KN0TPNA

Cloth Diaper 6pcs Pack
http://amzn.com/B00MFVNHXO